DIVERTICULITIS DIET FOR BEGINNERS

Unlock The Power Of Nutrient-Rich Foods To Optimize Digestive Health, Alleviate Symptoms, Rediscover Wellness, And Thrive In The Face Of Diverticulitis Challenges

DR. JACE ZAYDEN

Table of Contents

DISCLAIMER

The information provided in the book is intended for general informational purposes only. The content of this book should not be considered a substitute for professional medical advice, diagnosis, or treatment.

Readers are advised to consult with a qualified healthcare professional for medical advice tailored to their individual circumstances.

The author has made every effort to ensure that the information in this book is accurate and up-to-date at the time of publication. However, medical knowledge is constantly evolving, and new research may emerge that could impact the information presented. The author disclaims any responsibility for any adverse effects or consequences resulting from the use of the information provided in this book.

References or mentions of individuals, products, websites, organizations, or other names within this book are for informational purposes only and do not constitute an endorsement. The author has no affiliations with, and makes no endorsements of, any third-party entities mentioned. Readers are encouraged to conduct their own research and exercise their judgment when considering any external resources or recommendations.

The author and the publisher shall have neither liability nor responsibility to any person or entity with respect to any loss, damage, or injury caused or alleged to be caused directly or indirectly by the information contained in this book. Any reliance on the information within this book is at the reader's own risk.

By reading this book, the reader acknowledges and agrees to the terms of this disclaimer. If the reader does not agree with these terms, they should not use the information provided in this book.

ABOUT THIS BOOK

This book "Diverticulitis Diet" provides a comprehensive guide to managing the condition of diverticulitis through dietary choices, making it an indispensable resource for those afflicted with this condition. This book establishes the foundation by explicating the characteristics of diverticulitis in the introduction, thereby furnishing readers with a comprehensive comprehension of the condition. The causes, risk factors, and symptoms of diverticulitis, along with a thorough examination of medical treatment regimens and diagnostic procedures, are covered in detail in the next chapters. The primary emphasis of this book, nevertheless, is on the pivotal significance of diet in alleviating the symptoms of diverticulitis.

This book consistently emphasizes the importance of integrating dietary strategies, providing general guidelines, specific foods to incorporate, and others to avoid.

A sample diet plan for individuals with diverticulitis is provided, which offers practical advice on meal structures. Additionally, this book explores the critical significance of fiber and hydration, expanding on their advantageous effects in the management of diverticulitis. This book explores the concepts of meal planning and portion control to equip readers with practical strategies for constructing a nutritious and balanced diet.

In addition to discussing dietary considerations, this book delves into lifestyle adjustments, acknowledging the interdependence that exists between routine activities and the management of diverticulitis. As part of an ongoing process, monitoring and adjusting one's diet is described in detail. An entire section devoted to precautions and factors to be considered underscores the importance of adopting a comprehensive approach to health. This book culminates in a robust endorsement of seeking guidance from healthcare professionals, emphasizing the necessity of a collaborative endeavor to ensure the successful management of diverticulitis. Fundamentally, the "Diverticulitis Diet" functions as an indispensable manual, integrating scientific knowledge with pragmatic counsel, enabling individuals to effectively manage and alleviate the difficulties presented by diverticulitis by making well-informed dietary selections.

CHAPTER ONE

An Overview Of The Diverticulitis Diet:
Diverticulitis is a pathological state distinguished by the infection or inflammation of diverticula, which are diminutive cavities that may form along the intestinal mucosa, specifically in the large intestine. Although the precise etiology of diverticulitis remains unknown, there is a consensus that it is linked to a low-fiber dietary pattern. Consequently, dietary adjustments are of paramount importance in the prevention and management of diverticulitis. This book thoroughly examines diverticulitis, including its definition, etiology, clinical manifestations, and notably, the significance of adhering to a specialized diet designed for this condition.

Definition Of Diverticulitis

Diverticulitis is a pathological state characterized by the inflammation or infection of diverticula, which are diminutive protruding cavities that may develop in the intestinal mucosa, specifically in the colon.

As individuals age, diverticula, which are cavities, become more prevalent. Diverticulitis results from inflammation or infection of the diverticles and is characterized by a spectrum of symptoms including but not limited to severe pain, abdominal tenderness, fever, and alterations in bowel movements.

Diverticula development is frequently correlated with a low-fiber diet. The consumption of fiber is critical for the maintenance of digestive system health, the promotion of regular bowel movements, and the prevention of diverticula formation. Insufficient fiber in one's diet may lead to constipation, elevated colonic pressure, and the development of these pouches.

Due to the close association between diverticulitis and dietary factors, the implementation of a diverticulitis diet becomes crucial in its management.

Contributing Factors And Risk Elements

Although the exact etiology of diverticulitis remains unknown, specific risk factors and contributing elements have been identified. The main risk factor is consuming insufficient fiber. By increasing stool volume, fiber facilitates refuse movement through the digestive tract. Insufficient fiber intake results in rigid and difficult-to-move stools, which in turn increases the pressure on the walls of the colon. Diverticula may form as a result of the increased pressure.

Aging is another risk factor to consider, as it correlates with an increased likelihood of developing diverticulitis. Diverticular disease susceptibility may be increased in individuals with a familial predisposition to the condition, suggesting that genetics may also be a factor. Furthermore, specific medications, including nonsteroidal anti-inflammatory medicines (NSAIDs), obesity, and a sedentary lifestyle have been associated with an elevated likelihood of developing diverticulitis.

Recognizing these risk factors emphasizes the necessity of adopting a comprehensive strategy for managing diverticulitis, wherein dietary adjustments constitute its fundamental component. The primary objectives of a diverticulitis diet are symptom relief, prevention of inflammation, and promotion of digestive health.

Manifestations Of Diverticulitis

Diverticulitis is characterized by a range of symptoms, some of which may include abdominal tenderness, bloating, fever, nausea, vomiting, alterations in bowel movements, and pain in the lower left region of the abdomen. Complications such as colon perforation or abscess formation may arise in certain instances, resulting in the manifestation of more severe symptoms that necessitate immediate medical intervention.

The occurrence of symptoms frequently motivates people to pursue medical intervention. Imaging studies, including computed tomography (CT) scans, physical examination, and medical history are commonly utilized in the diagnostic process. Following a diagnosis, the treatment of diverticulitis frequently necessitates a comprehensive strategy, with diet being an essential component.

The Diverticulitis Diet: An Essential Component Of Treatment

The purpose of a diverticulitis diet is to target the underlying causes and manifestations of the condition. The principal emphasis is on augmenting the consumption of dietary fiber, given its capacity to supplement stool bulk, facilitate consistent bowel movements, and avert constipation. Vegetables, fruits, whole grains, legumes, and whole grains are all high in fiber. Gradual fiber incorporation is imperative to facilitate the digestive system's adaptation.

Apart from enhancing fiber intake, additional dietary modifications may be incorporated into the diverticulitis diet. For example, individuals diagnosed with diverticulitis may receive recommendations to abstain from including almonds, seeds, and popcorn, as these foods have the potential to exacerbate symptoms. While nuts and seeds have traditionally been considered problematic foods, recent research has called into doubt the advisability of strictly avoiding them.

Additionally, adequate hydration is vital for the management of diverticulitis. Adequate hydration facilitates bowel movement and aids in the prevention of constipation. It is advisable to ensure sufficient consumption of water, while alcohol and caffeinated beverages ought to be consumed in moderation.

In summary, diverticulitis is a medical condition that requires a holistic approach to treatment, wherein dietary adjustments are of paramount importance.

In addition to alleviating symptoms, a personalized diet abundant in fiber and designed to address specific dietary requirements can effectively avert the reoccurrence of diverticulitis. This highlights the importance of embracing a nutritious diet and maintaining a healthy lifestyle to ensure the digestive system's long-term health. Like any other medical condition, it is advisable for individuals diagnosed with diverticulitis to seek personalized advice and guidance from healthcare professionals regarding dietary choices.

Medical Evaluation And Management

Diverticulitis is a pathological state distinguished by the infection or inflammation of diverticula, which are diminutive cavities that may form along the intestinal mucosa, predominantly in the colon. In many cases, diverticulitis is diagnosed following a comprehensive physical examination and medical history review. Manifestations including fever, abdominal pain, and alterations in bowel movements may warrant additional examination.

Diagnostic instruments such as imaging studies (e.g., CT scans), blood tests, and colonoscopies are frequently utilized by medical professionals to ascertain the existence and extent of diverticulitis. The medical treatment approach is contingent upon the severity of the condition after its diagnosis. Antibiotics, painkillers, and a transient transition to a liquid or low-fiber diet may be employed to manage mild instances while the digestive tract recovers.

In cases of greater severity, hospitalization might be required. Antibiotics can be administered intravenously (IV), and in uncommon instances, surgical intervention or the drainage of abscesses may be necessary. In the majority of cases, diverticulitis is treated surgically, except in the case of recurrent episodes or complicated cases that do not respond to alternative therapies.

CHAPTER TWO

Dietary Importance In The Management Of Diverticulitis

The significance of diet in the management of diverticulitis is critical. Although diet may not be the exclusive determinant of diverticulitis, it can have a substantial influence on flare-up prevention and the overall management of the condition. A diet that is conducive to diverticulitis ought to decrease inflammation, encourage consistent gastrointestinal movements, and avert potential complications.

To manage diverticulitis, it is crucial to adhere to a sufficient dietary fiber regimen. The promotion of regular bowel movements and the prevention of constipation, both of which can contribute to the development of diverticula, are both dependent on fiber.

In addition, a diet rich in fiber may reduce colon inflammation and the likelihood of developing complications from diverticulitis.

1. Progressive Fiber Intake: Individuals diagnosed with diverticulitis must increase their fiber consumption progressively. Increases in fiber consumption that occur abruptly may result in flatulence, bloating, and discomfort. It is recommended to commence with soluble fiber sources that are readily digestible, such as those found in fruits and vegetables. Gradually integrate more insoluble fiber, such as that found in whole cereals and bran.

2. Sufficient Hydration: It is particularly critical to maintain an adequate water intake when augmenting fiber consumption. By absorbing water, fiber contributes to the bulk of the stool and facilitates its transit through the digestive tract. Optimal hydration is a critical component in the management of diverticulitis as it serves to prevent constipation.

3. Implementing Dietary Restrictions: Certain foods have the potential to worsen symptoms of diverticulitis. It is common for individuals to

receive recommendations to restrict or abstain from specific food items, including almonds, seeds, and popcorn, due to historical beliefs that linked them to diverticulitis. Recent research, nevertheless, indicates that these limitations might not be as essential as was previously believed. A healthcare professional can be of assistance in identifying dietary intolerances on an individual basis.

4. Consuming consistent, nutritionally balanced meals regularly can aid in the regulation of gastrointestinal movements and the promotion of digestive health as a whole. To prevent the digestive system from becoming overloaded, smaller, more frequent meals might be preferred over larger, less frequent ones.

Incorporating Foods Into A Diverticulitis Diet

1. A variety of fruits and vegetables that are rich in fiber should be incorporated into one's dietary regimen. Spinach, apples, pears, berries, broccoli, and carrots are all outstanding options. These

dietary items are rich in soluble fiber, vitamins, and minerals, which are all vital for maintaining optimal digestive health.

2. When making food choices, choose whole cereals such as quinoa, brown rice, and whole wheat bread. These cereals contribute to a balanced diet by facilitating regular gastrointestinal movements and being abundant in insoluble fiber.

3. Lean Protein: Incorporate into your meals lean protein sources such as poultry, fish, eggs, and tofu. Protein is vital for overall health and tissue repair. Select culinary techniques such as steaming, baking, or grilling to reduce the amount of oil added.

4. Foods Rich in Probiotics are advantageous bacteria that promote digestive health. Fermented vegetables, kefir, and yogurt containing live cultures are examples of foods that can introduce beneficial microbes into the digestive tract.

5. Selection of Healthful Fats: Opt for nutritious fat sources, including avocados, olive oil, and almonds. These lipids can supply vital nutrients while avoiding any inflammatory effects.

In conclusion, diverticulitis management necessitates a comprehensive strategy, in which diet assumes a critical component. Adhering to appropriate dietary selections can effectively mitigate symptoms, avert exacerbations, and promote holistic digestive health. Collaborating closely with healthcare professionals, such as registered dietitians, is imperative for individuals diagnosed with diverticulitis to customize their diet to specific requirements and guarantee a well-rounded and nourishing strategy for managing this condition.

A List Of Foods To Prevent Diverticulitis

Diverticulitis is a pathological state distinguished by the inflammatory formation of diverticula, which are diminutive cavities that may develop in the intestinal mucosa, specifically in the colon. Dietary modifications are frequently required to alleviate symptoms and prevent flare-ups of diverticulitis. People with diverticulitis must be aware of which foods should be avoided to prevent the condition from worsening.

1. Nuts and seeds are considered to be a significant contributor to flare-ups of diverticulitis. Trapped in the diverticula, these microscopic, rigid particulates may induce inflammation and irritation. For instance, peanuts, sunflower seeds, and popcorn ought to be precluded from one's dietary regimen.

2. High-Fiber Foods: Although fiber is generally advantageous for digestive health, it can pose a problem during an exacerbation of diverticulitis. Examples of such foods include specific fruits and vegetables and whole grains.

These foods have the potential to impede digestion and exacerbate symptoms. They are, nevertheless, typically reintroduced progressively once the inflammation has subsided.

3. Red meat, particularly meaty slices, has the potential to cause digestive distress. There is a possibility that the elevated fat content could induce inflammation and cause discomfort. For those with diverticulitis, reduced protein sources such as poultry, fish, or plant-based proteins may be preferable.

4. Dairy Products: Certain individuals diagnosed with diverticulitis may experience symptom onset in response to dairy products, especially those that are high in lipid content. Sensitivity to or intolerance to lactose may worsen digestive issues. As an alternative, selecting low-fat or lactose-free dairy products may be acceptable.

5. Spicy Foods: In patients with diverticulitis, spices and spicy peppers may cause increased inflammation and irritation of the digestive tract. Avoiding overly piquant foods is recommended to prevent discomfort and symptom exacerbation.

6. Processed foods frequently comprise detrimental lipids, additives, and preservatives,

all of which have the potential to exacerbate digestive problems. Individuals with diverticulitis should limit their consumption of processed munchies, canned products, and pre-packaged meals.

7. Both caffeine and alcohol have the potential to cause dehydration, which is not a healthy condition for those who have diverticulitis. Furthermore, these substances have the potential to cause discomfort by irritating the digestive tract. It is recommended to restrict or abstain from drinkable beverages that contain alcohol or caffeine.

8. Specific Carbohydrates and Fruits: Although fruits and vegetables are generally recommended for promoting a healthy diet, certain high-fiber options may require restriction when diverticulitis is at its worst. Raw vegetables, cruciferous vegetables (such as cauliflower and broccoli), and specific fruits that possess stiff coverings or seeds may present potential health hazards.

By avoiding these trigger foods from one's diet, diverticulitis symptoms can be better managed and the likelihood of flare-ups decreased. Nevertheless, it is critical to seek guidance from a healthcare professional or a registered dietitian to develop an individualized strategy that takes into account the specific requirements and gravity of the ailment.

CHAPTER THREE

A Diverticulitis Diet Plan Example

Diverticulitis sufferers must prioritize the development of a nutritious and well-balanced diet. A meticulously planned dietary regimen has the potential to mitigate symptoms, foster recovery, and avert recurrences. The following is an example of a diet plan for diverticulitis that emphasizes soft, readily digestible foods:

For breakfast,

• Oatmeal prepared with lactose-free milk or water

Slicing the banana

• Eggs scrambled

The midmorning snack consists of:

• Greek yogurt (lactose-free or low-fat)

• Ripe, tender berries, such as strawberries or blueberries

Dish for Lunch:

• Breast of grilled poultry

• White steamed rice

• Carrots and zucchini both cooked

Mashed potatoes (Mash)

Snack to Follow:

• Low-fat yogurt, banana, and a sprinkling of spinach blended into a smoothie

Saltine wafers (2)

Meal: Dinner

• Grilled or baked fish (such as tilapia or salmon)

Quinoa, a

Steamed green beans are the source.

Peeled and cooked sweet potatoes

Concluding Snack:

Apple sauce (2)

• Almond butter (with restraint)

Hydration And Its Function

Adequate hydration is an essential component in the management of diverticulitis. Adequate hydration is crucial for maintaining digestive health and averting constipation, which is frequently encountered among those diagnosed with diverticulitis. The following explains the importance of hydration and how to maintain it:

1. Prevention of Constipation: Diverticulitis symptoms may be exacerbated by constipation caused by inadequate water intake. Sufficient hydration facilitates bowel movements by softening diarrhea, thereby reducing the likelihood of complications.

2. Water is an essential component in facilitating digestion and nutrient absorption. It facilitates the digestion of food, enabling the body to extract

vital nutrients and enhancing digestive health as a whole.

3. Hydration is a critical component in the process of eliminating impurities from the body. Adequate water consumption aids the kidneys in the filtration of waste products, thereby preventing the accumulation of detrimental substances that may worsen the symptoms of diverticulitis.

4. Ensuring Mucous Membrane Integrity: For optimal functionality, the mucous membranes lining the digestive tract necessitate sufficient hydration.

Adequately hydrated mucous membranes reduce the risk of irritation and inflammation while protecting the intestinal mucosa.

It is imperative for individuals diagnosed with diverticulitis to consume copious amounts of water daily to maintain adequate hydration. Although it is generally advised to drink a minimum of eight 8-ounce containers of water per day, this may differ for individuals. Climate, level of physical activity, and general health should all be considered when calculating hydration needs.

It is crucial to acknowledge that although water serves as the principal hydration source, diluted fruit beverages and herbal infusions can also contribute to the total fluid intake.

On the contrary, moderate consumption of caffeinated and alcoholic beverages is advised as a result of their capacity to cause dehydration in the body.

Sustaining adequate hydration is a straightforward yet efficacious approach to managing diverticulitis and fostering digestive health as a whole.

Fiber And Its Advantages

Integrating fiber into a diverticulitis diet is of the utmost importance, as it promotes digestive health and prevents flare-ups. Although it may be necessary to restrict the consumption of high-fiber foods during acute episodes of diverticulitis, there are several advantages to reintroducing fiber progressively into the diet during periods of remission:

1. Preventing Constipation: By adding substance to diarrhea, insoluble fiber facilitates bowel movements and prevents constipation. It is especially critical for those who have diverticulitis, as constipation may exacerbate pressure in the colon, which could ultimately result in the development of diverticula.

2. Facilitation of Bowel Regularity: By fostering regularity, fiber aids in the regulation of bowel movements. Particularly advantageous are those afflicted with diverticulitis who may manifest irregular defecation patterns.

3. The maintenance of colon health is facilitated through the consumption of sufficient fiber, which promotes the proliferation of advantageous microbes and preserves a harmonious

microbiome. A colon in good health is less prone to developing diverticula and inflammation.

4. Blood Sugar Stabilization: Soluble fiber, which is present in fruits, legumes, and cereals, aids in the regulation of blood sugar levels. This is crucial for patients diagnosed with diverticulitis, as hyperglycemia has the potential to exacerbate the inflammatory response.

5. Weight Management: Foods that are rich in fiber typically contain fewer calories and promote satiety, both of which contribute to effective weight management. Sustaining a healthy weight is imperative for optimal general health and may aid in the mitigation of complications associated with diverticulitis.

To enhance fiber intake, it is advisable for individuals to progressively reintroduce foods that are rich in fiber during phases of remission. In addition to fruits and vegetables, whole cereals and legumes are also rich in fiber. Alongside a high-fiber diet, it is essential to consume copious amounts of water to facilitate the fiber's passage through the digestive tract.

Although fiber is generally advantageous, it is critical to devise an individualized plan in consultation with a registered dietitian or healthcare professional, taking into account specific dietary requirements and the stage of diverticulitis. By incorporating fiber gradually into their diet, individuals with diverticulitis can benefit from the many advantages of fiber without experiencing an exacerbation of symptoms during flare-ups.

CHAPTER FOUR

Meal Preparation And Portion Management In The Diverticulitis Diet

Diverticulitis, an intestinal disorder distinguished by the infection or inflammation of minor cavities lining the colon's walls, frequently requires dietary modifications for symptom control and the enhancement of general well-being. The implementation of meal planning and portion control is crucial when developing a diet that is considerate of diverticulitis and serves to mitigate symptoms and avert exacerbations.

Meal Preparation:

1. A high-fiber foundation is an essential component of a diet for diverticulitis. Fiber aids in the maintenance of regular bowel movements and prevents constipation, a frequent etiology of the condition. Legumes, fruits, whole cereals, and vegetables are all rich in dietary fiber. Whole-grain bread, brown rice, quinoa, and oats are all viable options for incorporating into dishes.

2. Lean proteins offer vital nutrients while avoiding an excessive amount of fat. Legumes, skinless poultry, fish, and tofu are all fantastic sources of protein. These alternatives reduce the likelihood that diverticulitis symptoms will worsen.

3. Include probiotic-rich foods in your diet, such as fermented vegetables, yogurt, and kefir. By encouraging the proliferation of beneficial bacteria, probiotics potentially mitigate inflammation in the colon, thereby promoting digestive health.

4. It is critical to maintain sufficient hydration to effectively manage diverticulitis. Water facilitates the elimination of impurities, prevents constipation, and aids in digestion. Aim for a minimum of eight glasses of water daily, increasing as necessary in response to activity levels and personal requirements.

Control of Portion:

1. It is crucial for individuals with diverticulitis to adhere to the principle of moderation by ingesting meals in moderate portions. Excessive food consumption can potentially strain the digestive system and elicit symptoms. By utilizing smaller plates and consuming more leisurely, one can more precisely measure portions.

2. Balanced Meals: Aim to incorporate a variety of nutrients into your meals, including fiber, protein, healthy lipids, and carbohydrates. This equilibrium guarantees continuous energy levels and promotes general well-being.

3. Consistent, Smaller Meals: Opt for distributing food consumption across five to six smaller meals over the course of the day, as opposed to three substantial meals. This methodology has the potential to mitigate the risk of digestive system excess and enhance symptom management efficacy.

4. Eating mindfully requires paying close attention to appetite and satiety indicators. Savoring each mouthful, chewing thoroughly, and recognizing when one is comfortably filled are all components of mindful dining. This practice has the potential to decrease the likelihood of excess and enhance digestion.

Lifestyle Modifications For The Management Of Diverticulitis

In addition to meal planning, the management of diverticulitis can be substantially improved by incorporating specific lifestyle adjustments that effectively alleviate symptoms and enhance overall health.

1. Participating in consistent physical activity is advantageous in the management of diverticulitis. Physical activity enhances colon health by reducing inflammation and promoting regularity of the bowel. Most days of the week, strive to complete at least 30 minutes of moderate exercise, such as vigorous walking.

2. Stress Reduction Strategies: The symptoms of diverticulitis may be worsened by chronic stress. Integrate daily mindfulness practices, meditation, deep breathing exercises, or yoga into your regimen as stress-reduction strategies. These practices may have a beneficial effect on digestive health and stress management.

3. Preventing Trigger Food Ingestion: Recognize and abstain from consuming foods that have the potential to induce flare-ups of diverticulitis. Spicy foods, high-fat products, and specific seeds or legumes are frequently detected as triggers. Maintaining a food diary can assist in identifying particular triggers and shaping dietary decisions.

4. Establishing regular gastrointestinal habits is an essential component in the management of diverticulitis. Consistent and punctual bowel movements reduce the likelihood of developing diverticulitis-causing constipation. People must satisfy their natural impulses without delay, including defecation.

Observing And Modifying The Diet

Constant monitoring of the diet for diverticulitis is critical to accommodate evolving requirements and reduce the likelihood of symptom recurrence.

1. Symptom Pattern Observation: Maintain a close watch on how various substances affect your symptoms. Observe any recurring patterns or precipitating factors that could result in exacerbations. This consciousness enables prompt modifications to the dietary regimen.

2. Gradual Reintroduction of Foods: Once symptoms have been effectively managed, contemplate the gradual reintroduction of specific foods that were initially restricted. Observe the body's response and make necessary dietary adjustments. A systematic progression can facilitate the identification of particular inclinations and tolerances.

3. Seeking the Advice of a Registered Dietitian: Precise advice can be obtained from a registered dietitian who specializes in gastrointestinal

health. In addition to evaluating dietary patterns, addressing nutrient deficiencies, and providing personalized recommendations for the most effective management of diverticulitis, they are capable of doing so.

4. It is important to maintain proper hydration levels by consuming sufficient fluids and making adjustments according to factors such as activity levels, climate, and individual requirements. Constipation may be exacerbated by dehydration, which may also result in the onset of diverticulitis symptoms.

Considerations And Precautions

Diverticulitis patients must observe specific precautions and take into account particular factors to maintain the efficacy of dietary and lifestyle adjustments.

1. Caffeine and Alcohol Restrictions: Alcohol and caffeine overdose can irritate the digestive tract. Caffeinated and alcoholic beverages, including

coffee and tea, should be consumed in moderation to aid in symptom management.

2. Medication management may be recommended for individuals diagnosed with diverticulitis to alleviate symptoms. Adherence to medication regimens prescribed by healthcare professionals and timely communication of any concerns or adverse effects are of utmost importance.

3. Consistent Medical Examinations: Establish a routine for consultations with healthcare professionals to assess the comprehensive efficacy of diverticulitis treatment. This facilitates prompt modifications to the treatment regimen in response to changing health requirements.

4. Personalized Approach: Acknowledge the potential variability in an individual's response to strategies for managing diverticulitis. Adapt dietary and lifestyle adjustments to the specific symptom patterns, preferences, and tolerances of each individual.

Professional Consultation In The Healthcare Field

Seeking guidance from healthcare professionals is essential for the successful management of diverticulitis, as it guarantees a thorough and personalized approach.

1. It is advisable to maintain routine consultations with a primary care physician or gastroenterologist to monitor diverticulitis symptoms and conduct an overall health assessment. These experts are capable of offering counsel regarding the administration of medications and possible interventions.

2. Engage in a collaborative effort with a registered dietitian who possesses expertise in the field of gastrointestinal health. In addition to conducting comprehensive assessments, dietitians also offer individualized dietary recommendations and continuous support to facilitate long-term management.

3. The monitoring and modification of treatment plans are critical responsibilities of healthcare

professionals in the context of diverticulitis. They possess the ability to modify medications, suggest supplementary interventions, and verify that the comprehensive care strategy is on the personal health objectives of the individual.

4. Emergency Preparedness: Individuals must possess knowledge of emergency protocols in case they experience severe symptoms or complications.

When it is critical to seek immediate medical attention, acute diverticulitis episodes must be managed.

In summary, a meticulously organized diet for diverticulitis, which includes elements such as meal preparation, portion regulation, adjustments to one's lifestyle, and ongoing supervision, functions as a fundamental element in the successful management of symptoms? Consistent consultation with healthcare professionals, precautionary measures, and thoughtful considerations serve to augment the overall approach, enabling individuals to live healthier lives under control of their symptoms.

Conclusion

In summary, it is critical to adhere to a balanced and high-fiber diet to effectively manage diverticulitis and mitigate the risk of its reoccurrence. The underlying tenet of a diverticulitis diet is to facilitate digestive health by reducing the burden on the colon. Adequate consumption of soluble and insoluble fiber facilitates the maintenance of regular bowel movements, the prevention of constipation, and the reduction of colon pressure.

Additionally, the ingestion of probiotics, which are present in fermented foods and yogurt, may promote healthy intestinal microbiota, thereby enhancing the functionality of the immune system and potentially mitigating the symptoms linked to diverticulitis. Hydration is of equal importance, as it facilitates the passage of excrement and supports overall digestive function.

It is essential to adhere to a diet that is suitable for individuals with diverticulitis; however, for tailored guidance, it is critical to seek the opinion of a healthcare professional. The degree to which individuals react to dietary modifications can differ, and medical advice can assist in customizing dietary suggestions to account for particular circumstances and requirements.

Fundamentally, adopting a diverticulitis diet represents a sustainable lifestyle choice rather than a transient expedient. By placing dietary modifications as a top priority, individuals can proactively manage diverticulitis, improve their digestive health, and foster sustained gastrointestinal well-being.

THE END